CHAIR YOGA FOR WOMEN OVER 40

The Complete Guide to Transform Your Health, Renew Your Energy, and Achieve Inner Balance

MARTINE J. TOLEDO

Copyright © 2024 by MARTINE J. TOLEDO

TABLE OF CONTENT

INTRODUCTION

Lisa, a woman in her late forties, had always been content with her life. She had a steady job, a loving family, and a few close friends. However, she couldn't shake off the feeling that something was missing. She had been feeling increasingly restless and disconnected from her own body.

One day, as she was browsing through the shelves of a local bookstore, her eyes landed on a book titled "Chair Yoga for Women over 40." Intrigued, she picked it up and started flipping through its pages. The book promised to bring balance, harmony, and rejuvenation to one's life through the practice of gentle yoga exercises specifically designed for those with physical limitations.

Lisa had never tried yoga before, but she felt an inexplicable pull towards the book. She purchased it and brought it home, unsure of what to expect. That evening, she curled up on her favorite armchair, opened the book, and began to read.

The author of the book, a seasoned yoga instructor named Maya, shared stories of women who had found incredible transformation through practicing chair yoga. Lisa read about women who had regained their strength, flexibility, and inner peace. She learned about how chair yoga could improve posture, relieve stress, and enhance overall well-being.

Intrigued and inspired, Lisa decided to give chair yoga a try. She followed the simple instructions in the book, starting with gentle stretches and breathing exercises. At first, she felt a bit self-conscious and awkward, but she persisted, trusting in the process.

As the days turned into weeks, Lisa began to notice subtle changes within herself. She found herself feeling more present in her body, more aware of her breathing, and more attuned to her inner self. The tension that had built up in her shoulders from hours of sitting at a desk started to melt away. Her body felt lighter, and her mind felt calmer.

Lisa's newfound sense of balance and tranquility started to permeate other areas of her life. She discovered that she had more patience and resilience in dealing with everyday challenges. She became more mindful of her eating habits and started incorporating healthier choices into her diet. The simple act of practicing chair yoga had sparked a positive ripple effect in her life.

One morning, as Lisa was engrossed in a challenging yoga pose from the book, her daughter walked into the room. Astonished by her mother's newfound flexibility and graceful movements, her daughter asked if she could join in. Lisa happily obliged, and soon enough, they were both practicing chair yoga together.

Word of Lisa's transformation spread among her friends and coworkers. They witnessed her vibrant energy, her radiance, and her newfound zest for life. Curiosity piqued, they, too, started exploring the world of chair yoga.

Lisa's journey with chair yoga had not only transformed her life but had also become a catalyst for positive change in the lives of those around her. The simple act of coming into contact with a book had set her on a path of self-discovery, healing, and connection.

As the years passed, Lisa continued to practice chair yoga, deepening her practice and sharing her knowledge with others. She became a certified chair yoga instructor and created a community of women over 40 who came together to support and uplift each other through their shared love for chair yoga.

Looking back on her journey, Lisa realized that sometimes, the most profound changes in life come from unexpected encounters. The book had been the catalyst that ignited her transformation, but it was her courage, determination, and open heart that had allowed her to embrace the change and grow into the best version of herself.

And so, Lisa's story serves as a reminder to all of us that change can come in the most unexpected ways, and sometimes, all it takes is a book, an open mind, and a willingness to embark on a journey of self-discovery.

EXERCISE

General Guidelines

Prepare Your Space:

- Find a quiet and comfortable space where you can practice chair yoga without distractions.
- Choose a sturdy chair without wheels, preferably with a straight back and no armrests.
- Ensure that there is enough room around you to move your arms and legs freely.

Warm-Up:

- Start with a few minutes of deep breathing to center yourself and prepare your body for the practice.
- Sit tall on the chair, close your eyes, and take slow, deep breaths in and out through your nose. Focus on relaxing any tension in your body with each exhale.

Gentle Stretches:

- Begin with gentle stretches to warm up your muscles and increase flexibility.

- Perform neck stretches by slowly tilting your head forward, backward, and sideways, being mindful of any discomfort.

- Stretch your shoulders by rolling them forward and backward and gently raise and lower them.

- Stretch your arms by reaching them overhead and then out to the sides, feeling a gentle stretch in your shoulders and upper back.

Seated Poses:

- Explore various seated yoga poses that promote strength, flexibility, and relaxation.

- Practice seated twists by placing your left hand on the outside of your right thigh and gently rotating your torso to the right. Repeat on the other side.

- Engage your core muscles by lifting one leg at a time, straightening it out in front of you, and holding for a few breaths. Lower it back down and repeat with the other leg.
- Stretch your hamstrings by extending one leg straight out and gently reaching towards your toes. Hold for a few breaths and switch legs.

Breathing Exercises:

- Incorporate pranayama (breathing exercises) to enhance relaxation and focus.
- Practice deep belly breathing by inhaling deeply through your nose, allowing your belly to expand, and exhaling slowly through your mouth.
- Try alternate nostril breathing by using your right thumb to close your right nostril, inhaling through your left nostril, then closing your left nostril with your right ring finger and exhaling through your right nostril. Repeat on the other side.

Mindfulness and Meditation:

- Dedicate a few minutes to quiet meditation or mindfulness practice to promote mental clarity and relaxation.
- Sit comfortably in your chair, close your eyes, and focus on your breath. Notice the sensation of the breath entering and leaving your body.
- Allow any thoughts or distractions to pass by without judgment, returning your attention to the present moment and the sensation of your breath.

Cool Down and Relaxation:

- Finish your chair yoga practice with a few minutes of gentle stretches and relaxation.
- Perform gentle shoulder rolls, neck stretches, and deep breathing to release any remaining tension.
- Close your practice by sitting quietly, feeling the support of the chair beneath you, and expressing gratitude for the time you've dedicated to yourself.

Mind-Body Connection:

- Emphasize the connection between your mind and body during chair yoga practice.
- Be mindful of each movement and stretch, focusing on the sensations and how they affect your body.
- Use your breath as a guide, inhaling deeply during stretches and exhaling to release any tension.

Enhance Stability and Balance:

- Improve your balance and stability by incorporating specific exercises into your chair yoga routine.
- Try seated leg lifts, gradually raising one leg at a time and holding it for a few seconds, then lowering it back down.
- Experiment with toe taps, gently tapping your toes on the floor while keeping your core engaged and your posture aligned.

Consistency and Self-Care:

- Make chair yoga a consistent part of your self-care routine to experience long-lasting benefits.
- Aim to practice chair yoga several times a week, gradually increasing the duration and complexity of your sessions.
- Take pleasure in your progress and be kind and patient with yourself, understanding that self-care is an ongoing journey unique to each individual.

Chair yoga offers a range of benefits specifically tailored to women over 40. Here are some key advantages:

Gentle and Safe: Chair yoga is a gentle and safe form of exercise, making it ideal for women over 40 who may have physical limitations or reduced mobility. It provides a low-impact option that minimizes strain on joints and muscles while still allowing for a beneficial workout.

Flexibility and Range of Motion: Regular chair yoga practice can improve flexibility and increase the range of motion in joints and muscles. The gentle stretches and movements help to release tension, reduce stiffness, and enhance overall physical comfort.

Strength and Balance: Chair yoga incorporates poses and exercises that target core muscles, arms, legs, and back. By engaging in these movements, women over 40 can strengthen their muscles, improve balance, and enhance overall stability, which is important for maintaining independence and reducing the risk of falls.

Stress Relief and Relaxation: Chair yoga includes breathing techniques and mindfulness practices that promote relaxation and stress reduction. Deep breathing exercises and guided meditation help women over 40 manage stress, improve mental well-being, and cultivate a sense of inner calm.

Posture and Spine Health: Chair yoga focuses on improving posture and spinal alignment. Regular practice can counteract the negative effects of prolonged sitting, leading to better spinal health and a reduced risk of back pain or discomfort commonly experienced by those with sedentary lifestyles.

Improved Circulation and Energy: The gentle movements and stretches in chair yoga stimulate blood circulation and energy flow throughout the body. This can lead to increased vitality, improved digestion, and an overall sense of well-being.

Mind-Body Connection: Chair yoga encourages a deeper mind-body connection by promoting awareness of sensations, breath, and movement. This enhances body awareness, self-compassion, and self-acceptance, fostering a positive attitude towards aging and self-care.

Social Connection and Support: Participating in chair yoga classes or group sessions provides an opportunity for women over 40 to connect with others who share similar interests and experiences. This fosters a sense of community, support, and social well-being.

It's important to remember that individual experiences may vary. If you have any pre-existing health conditions or concerns, it's recommended to consult with a healthcare professional before starting any exercise program, including chair yoga.

EXERCISE 1: SEATED CAT-COW POSE

Introduction:

The Seated Cat-Cow Pose is a gentle spinal movement that promotes flexibility and releases tension in the back.

Instructions:

- Sit upright on a chair with feet flat on the floor, hands resting on your thighs.
- Inhale deeply and arch your back, lifting your chest and bringing your shoulder blades together (Cow Pose).
- Exhale slowly, rounding your spine, tucking your chin to your chest, and drawing your navel in towards your spine (Cat Pose).
- Repeat this flowing movement, synchronizing it with your breath.

Benefits:

- Increases spinal mobility and flexibility.
- Relieves back pain and stiffness.
- Stimulates digestion and massages abdominal organs.

Image:

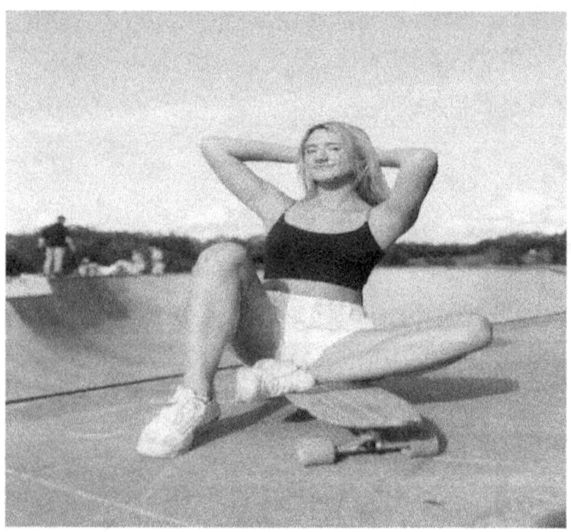

Sets and Repetitions:

Perform 3-5 sets, moving through the Cat-Cow sequence 5-8 times in each set.

EXERCISE 2: SEATED FORWARD FOLD

Introduction:

The Seated Forward Fold helps to stretch the hamstrings, lower back, and shoulders while promoting relaxation and calmness.

Instructions:

- Sit on the edge of the chair with your feet hip-width apart.
- Inhale deeply, lengthen your spine, and reach your arms overhead.
- Exhale slowly as you hinge forward from your hips, reaching your hands towards your feet or the floor.
- Relax your head and neck, allowing gravity to gently deepen the stretch.
- Hold the position for a few deep breaths.

Benefits:

- Stretches the back, hamstrings, and shoulders.
- Relieves tension and stress.
- Improves posture and spine health.

Image: 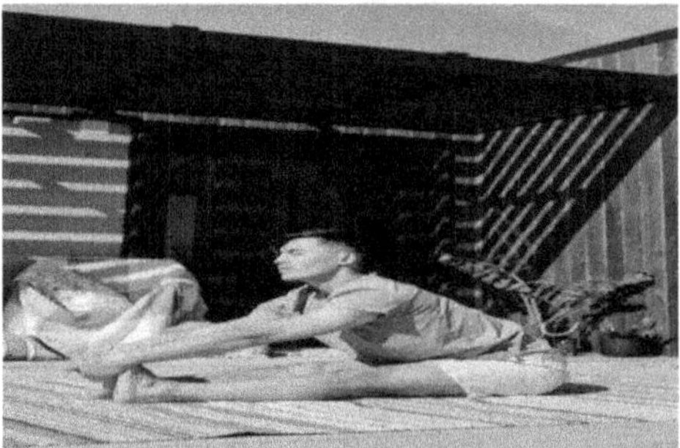

Sets and Repetitions: Hold the Seated Forward Fold for 3-5 breaths and repeat 3-5 times.

EXERCISE 3: SEATED SPINAL TWIST

Introduction:

The Seated Spinal Twist gently mobilizes the spine, improves digestion, and releases tension in the back and hips.

Instructions:

- Sit tall in the chair with your feet firmly planted on the ground.
- Inhale deeply, lengthen your spine, and place your left hand on the outside of your right thigh.
- Exhale slowly as you twist to the right, using your left hand to deepen the twist while placing your right hand on the back of the chair.
- Hold the twist for a few breaths, feeling the gentle rotation through your spine.
- Repeat the twist on the other side.

Benefits:

- Increases spinal mobility and flexibility.

- Relieves back pain and stiffness.

- Stimulates digestion and detoxification.

Image:

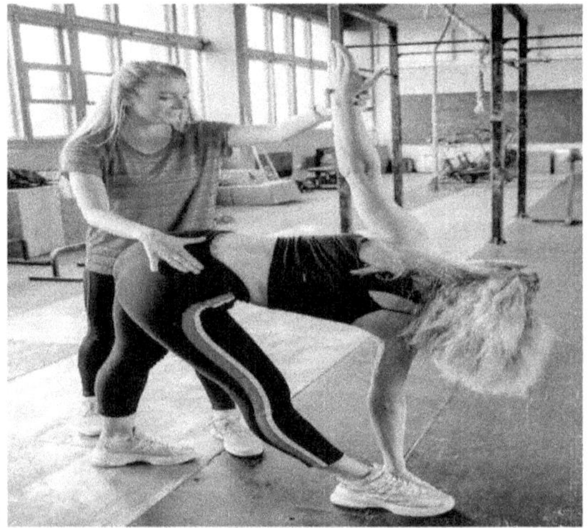

Sets and Repetitions:

Hold each side of the twist for 3-5 breaths and repeat 3-5 times on each side.

EXERCISE 4: SEATED LEG EXTENSIONS

Introduction:

Seated Leg Extensions strengthen the quadriceps, improve circulation, and enhance lower body strength and stability.

Instructions:

- ➤ Sit tall on the chair with your feet flat on the floor and hands resting on your thighs.
- ➤ Inhale deeply, engage your core, and extend your right leg straight out in front of you.
- ➤ Hold the position for a few seconds, flexing your foot and engaging your thigh muscles.
- ➤ Slowly lower your leg back down to the starting position.
- ➤ Repeat the movement with your left leg.

Benefits:

- ➢ Strengthens the quadriceps and improves lower body stability.
- ➢ Enhances circulation and reduces swelling in the legs.
- ➢ Improves balance and posture.

Image: 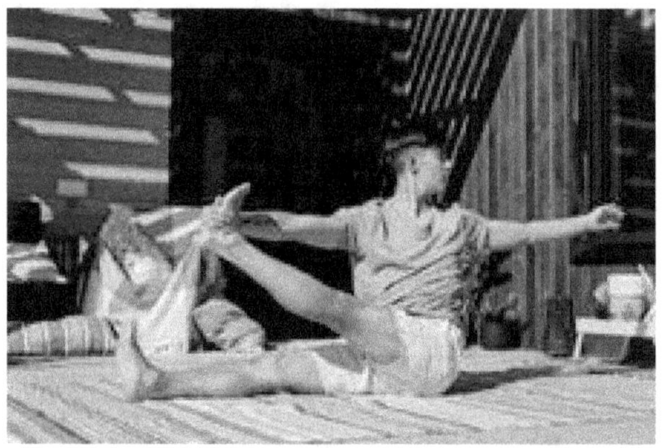

Sets and Repetitions:

Perform 2-3 sets of 10-12 leg extensions on each leg.

Exercise 5: Seated Shoulder Rolls

Introduction:

Seated Shoulder Rolls help release tension in the shoulders and upper back, improving posture and relieving neck and shoulder discomfort.

Instructions:

- ➢ Sit tall in the chair with your feet flat on the floor.
- ➢ Inhale deeply and lift your shoulders up towards your ears.
- ➢ Exhale slowly as you roll your shoulders back and down in a circular motion.
- ➢ Repeat the shoulder rolls in the opposite direction.

Benefits:

Releases tension and stiffness in the shoulders and upper back.

> ➢ Improves posture and alignment.
> ➢ Relieves neck and shoulder pain.

Image: 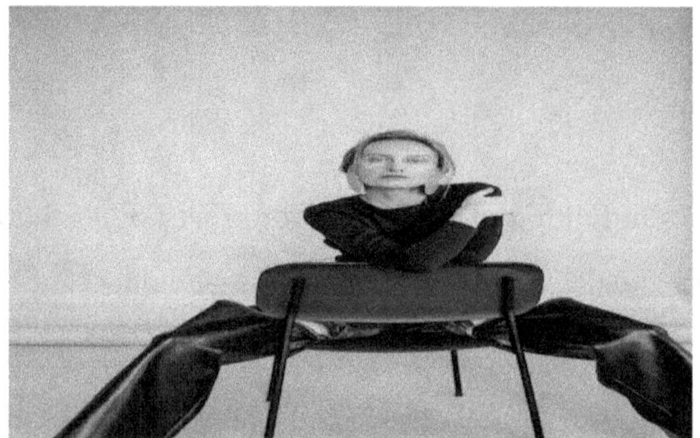

Sets and Repetitions:

Perform 2-3 sets of 8-10 shoulder rolls in each direction.

.

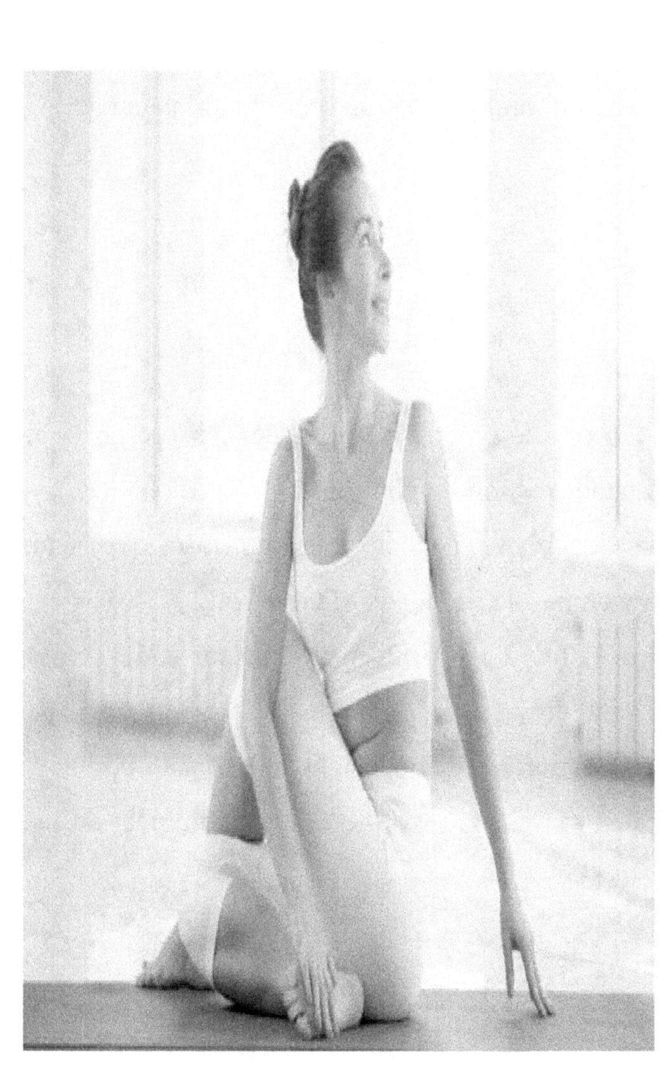

EXERCISE 6: SEATED SIDE BEND

Introduction:

The Seated Side Bend stretches the sides of the body, promotes spinal mobility, and enhances breathing capacity.

Instructions:

- ➤ Sit tall on the chair with your feet flat on the floor and hands resting on your thighs.
- ➤ Inhale deeply and reach your right arm overhead, lengthening the right side of your body.
- ➤ Exhale slowly as you lean to the left, sliding your left hand down your left thigh.
- ➤ Feel the stretch along the right side of your body.
- ➤ Inhale to come back to the center and repeat on the other side.

Benefits:

- Stretches the sides of the body and improves flexibility.
- Increases lung capacity and deepens breathing.
- Promotes spine health and mobility.

Image:

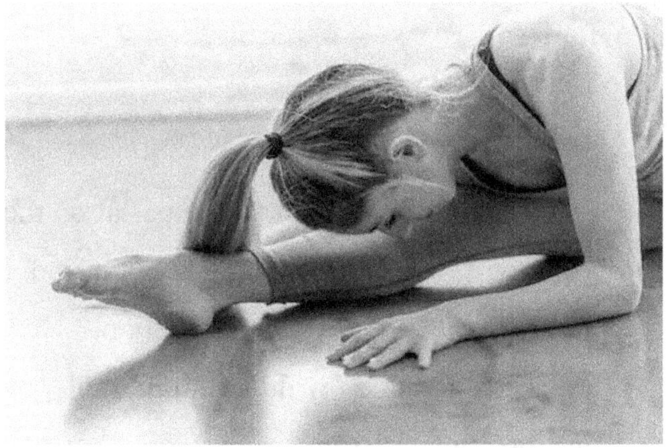

Sets and Repetitions:

Perform 3-5 sets on each side, holding the stretch for 3-5 deep breaths.

EXERCISE 7: SEATED ANKLE CIRCLES

Introduction:

Seated Ankle Circles increase ankle mobility, improve circulation in the lower extremities, and reduce stiffness.

Instructions:

- ➢ Sit tall on the chair with your feet flat on the floor.
- ➢ Lift your right foot off the ground and begin to rotate your ankle in a circular motion.
- ➢ Make the circles as wide as comfortable, moving in one direction.
- ➢ After a few rotations, switch to the opposite direction.
- ➢ Lower your right foot and repeat the circles with your left foot.

Benefits:

- ➢ Enhances ankle flexibility and range of motion.
- ➢ Stimulates blood flow and reduces swelling in the lower legs.
- ➢ Helps alleviate ankle and foot stiffness.

Image:
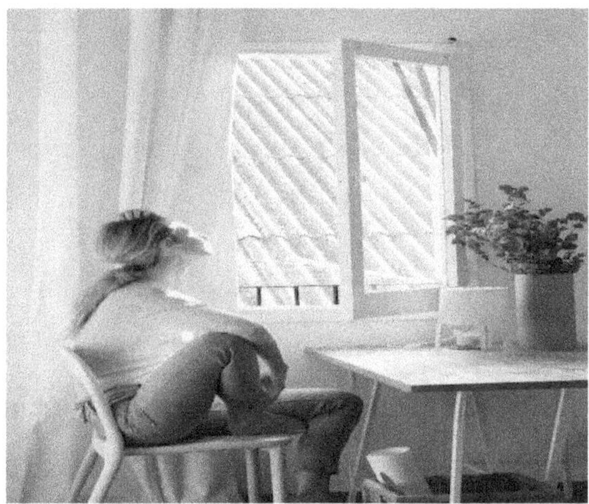

Sets and Repetitions:

Perform 2-3 sets of 8-10 ankle circles in each direction for each foot.

EXERCISE 8: SEATED CHEST OPENER

Introduction:

The Seated Chest Opener stretches the chest muscles, improves posture, and counteracts the effects of prolonged sitting.

Instructions:

- ➢ Sit tall on the chair with your feet flat on the floor and hands resting on your thighs.
- ➢ Inhale deeply, interlace your fingers behind your back, and squeeze your shoulder blades together.
- ➢ Exhale slowly as you gently lift your arms away from your back, opening your chest.
- ➢ Keep your chin slightly tucked to maintain alignment.
- ➢ Hold the stretch for a few deep breaths.

Benefits:

> ➢ Stretches the chest and shoulders, improving posture.
> ➢ Relieves tension in the upper back and neck.
> ➢ Enhances breathing capacity.

Image:

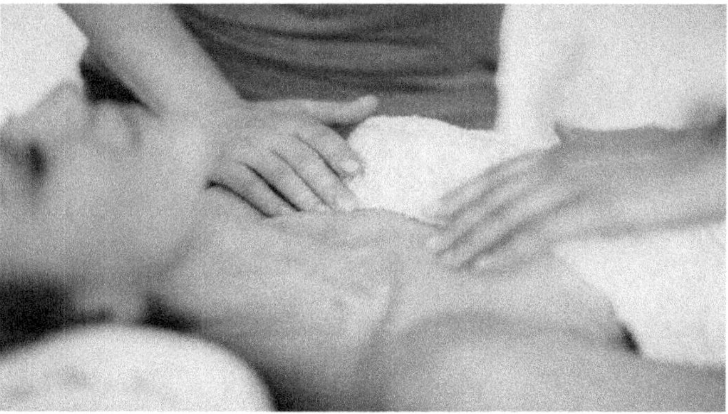

Sets and Repetitions:

Perform 3-5 sets, holding the stretch for 15-30 seconds in each set.

EXERCISE 9: SEATED LEG CROSS STRETCH

Introduction:

The Seated Leg Cross Stretch stretches the hips, glutes, and lower back, promoting flexibility and relieving tightness.

Instructions:

- Sit tall on the chair with your feet flat on the floor.
- Cross your right ankle over your left thigh, allowing your right knee to drop out to the side.
- Inhale deeply and lengthen your spine.
- Exhale slowly as you hinge forward from your hips, keeping your back straight.
- Feel the stretch in your right hip and glut.
- Hold the stretch for a few breaths, and then switch sides.

Benefits:

> ➢ Stretches the hips, gluts, and lower back.
>
> ➢ Relieves tightness and discomfort in the hip area.
>
> ➢ Improves flexibility and range of motion.

Image: 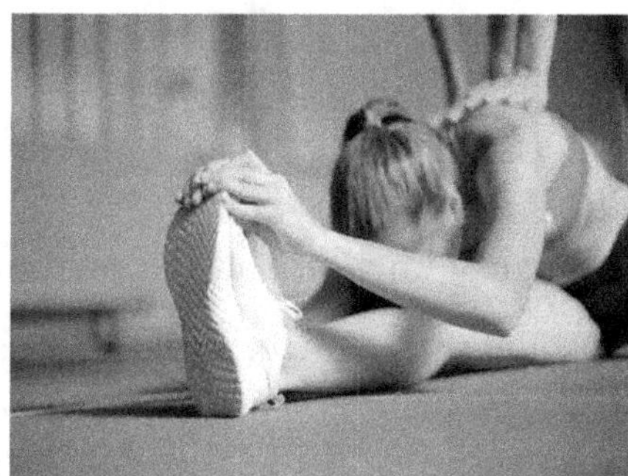

Sets and Repetitions:

Perform 2-3 sets on each side, holding the stretch for 20-30 seconds

.

EXERCISE 10: SEATED NECK ROLLS

Introduction:

Seated Neck Rolls release tension in the neck and shoulders, improve mobility, and promote relaxation.

Instructions:

- ➤ Sit tall on the chair with your feet flat on the floor.
- ➤ Inhale deeply, lengthen your spine, and relax your shoulders.
- ➤ Exhale slowly as you drop your right ear towards your right shoulder.
- ➤ Inhale to bring your head back to the center.
- ➤ Exhale as you drop your left ear towards your left shoulder.
- ➤ Continue to roll your neck gently from side to side.

Benefits:

> - Relieves tension and stiffness in the neck and shoulders.
> - Improves neck mobility and range of motion.
> - Promotes relaxation and stress relief.

Image:

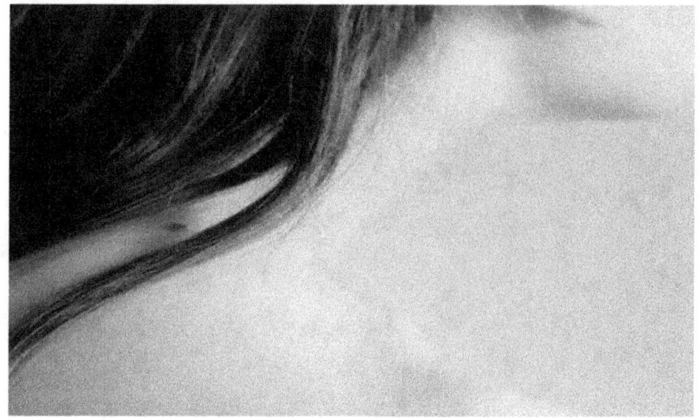

Sets and Repetitions:

Perform 2-3 sets, rolling the neck gently from side to side 8-10 times in each set.

Remember to listen to your body and adjust the exercises as needed. If you experience any pain or discomfort during the practice, please stop and consult with a healthcare professional. Enjoy your chair yoga routine!

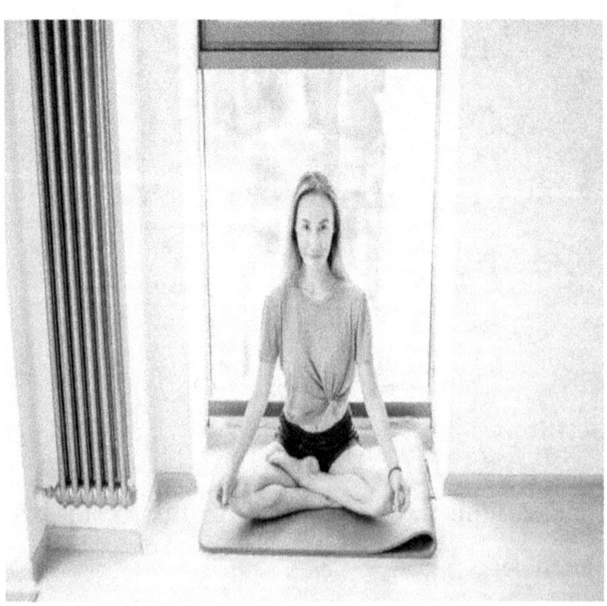

EXERCISE 11: SEATED LEG CROSS TWIST

Introduction:

The Seated Leg Cross Twist stretches the spine, hips, and shoulders, improving flexibility and releasing tension.

Instructions:

- ➢ Sit tall on the chair with your feet flat on the floor.
- ➢ Cross your right ankle over your left thigh, placing your right foot on the floor.
- ➢ Inhale deeply and lengthen your spine.
- ➢ Exhale slowly as you twist your torso to the right, placing your left hand on your right thigh for support.
- ➢ Gently twist from your waist, feeling the stretch in your spine and shoulders.
- ➢ Hold the twist for a few breaths, then switch sides.

Benefits:

- ➢ Stretches the spine, hips, and shoulders.
- ➢ Improves spinal mobility and posture.
- ➢ Relieves tension and tightness in the upper body.

Image:

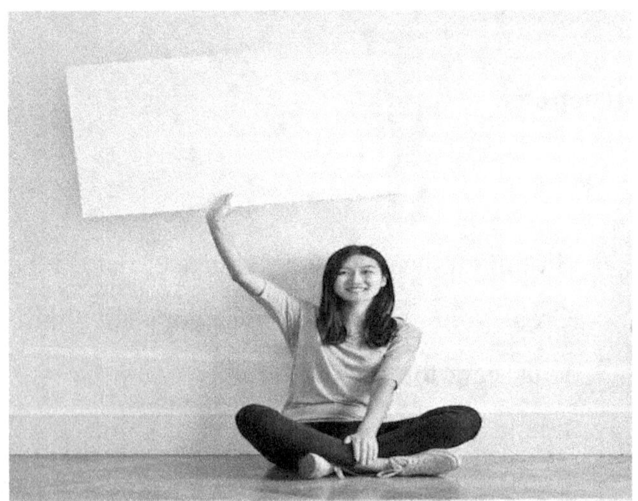

Sets and Repetitions:

Perform 3-5 sets on each side, holding the twist for 3-5 breaths.

EXERCISE 12: SEATED WRIST AND FINGER STRETCH

Introduction:

The Seated Wrist and Finger Stretch improves flexibility and relieves tension in the wrists and fingers, which can be beneficial for those who spend a lot of time typing or using handheld devices.

Instructions:

>
> Sit tall on the chair with your feet flat on the floor.
> Extend your arms straight in front of you at shoulder height.
> Spread your fingers wide apart.
> Slowly flex your wrists, pointing your fingers towards the ceiling.
> Hold the stretch for a few seconds, feeling the stretch in your wrists and fingers.
> Relax and return to the starting position.

> Repeat the stretch, this time extending your fingers towards the floor.

Benefits:

> Increases flexibility and range of motion in the wrists and fingers.
> Relieves tension and stiffness caused by repetitive hand movements.
> Enhances hand and finger dexterity.

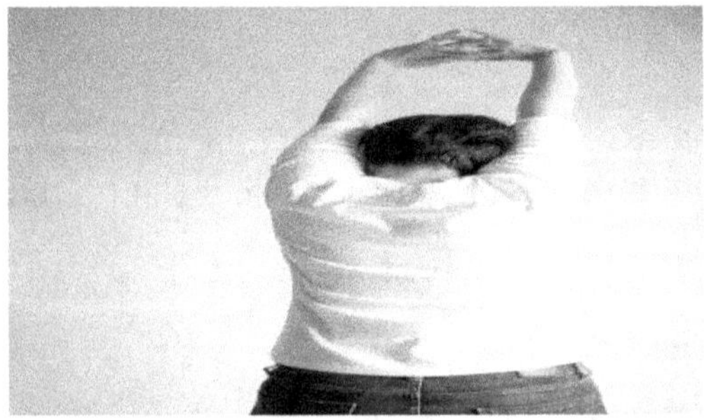

Image:

Sets and Repetitions:

Perform 2-3 sets, holding each stretch for 10-15 seconds in each set.

EXERCISE 13: SEATED HIP OPENER

Introduction:

The Seated Hip Opener stretches the hips, gluts, and inner thighs, promoting flexibility and reducing tightness.

Instructions:

- ➢ Sit tall on the chair with your feet flat on the floor.
- ➢ Place your right ankle on top of your left knee, allowing your right knee to drop out to the side.
- ➢ Inhale deeply and lengthen your spine.
- ➢ Exhale slowly as you hinge forward from your hips, maintaining a straight back.
- ➢ Feel the stretch in your right hip and outer thigh.
- ➢ Hold the stretch for a few breaths, then switch sides.

Benefits:

- ➢ Stretches the hips, gluts, and inner thighs.
- ➢ Relieves tightness and discomfort in the hip area.
- ➢ Improves hip flexibility and range of motion.

Image:

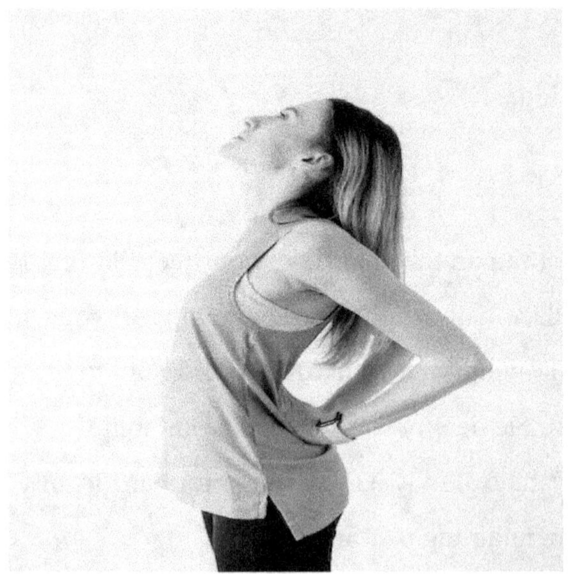

Sets and Repetitions:

Perform 2-3 sets on each side, holding the stretch for 20-30 seconds.

EXERCISE 14: SEATED EAGLE ARMS

Introduction:

Seated Eagle Arms stretch the shoulders, upper back, and arms, improving posture and releasing tension.

Instructions:

- ➢ Sit tall on the chair with your feet flat on the floor.
- ➢ Inhale deeply and extend your arms straight in front of you.
- ➢ Cross your right arm over your left arm at the elbows, bringing your palms to touch if possible.
- ➢ Lift your elbows slightly, feeling the stretch in your upper back and shoulders.
- ➢ Hold the position for a few breaths, then switch the crossing of your arms.
- ➢ Repeat the stretch on the other side.

Benefits:

> ➢ Stretches the shoulders, upper back, and arms.
>
> ➢ Improves posture and alignment.
>
> ➢ Relieves tension and tightness in the upper body.

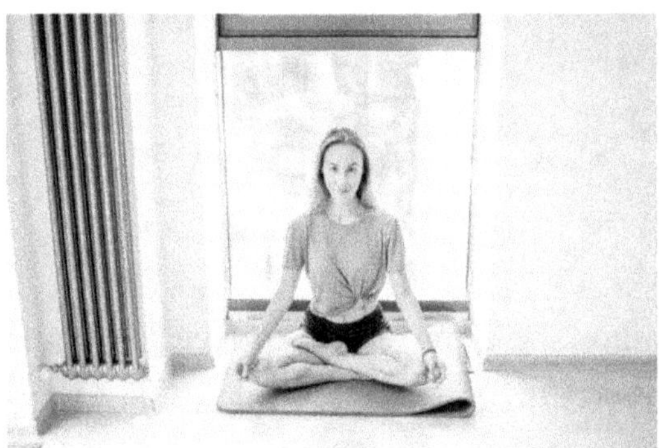

Image:

Sets and Repetitions:

Perform 3-5 sets, holding the stretch for 10-15 seconds in each set.

EXERCISE 15: SEATED ABDOMINAL TWIST

Introduction:

The Seated Abdominal Twist stretches the spine, improves digestion, and releases tension in the back and waist.

Instructions:

➢ Sit tall on the chair with your feet flat on the floor.

➢ Place your right hand on the outside of your left thigh.

➢ Inhale deeply, lengthen your spine, and sit tall.

➢ Exhale slowly as you twist your torso to the left, using your right hand to deepen the twist.

➢ Look over your left shoulder, feeling the stretch in your spine and waist.

Hold the twist for a few breaths, and then switch sides

Benefits:

- ➢ Stretches the spine, improving spinal mobility and flexibility.
- ➢ Aids in digestion and stimulates the abdominal organs.
- ➢ Relieves tension and tightness in the back and waist.

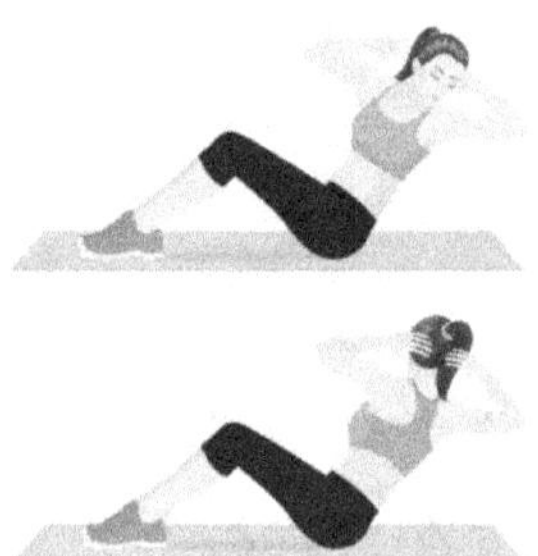

Image:

Sets and Repetitions:

Perform 3-5 sets on each side, holding the twist for 3-5 breaths.

Remember to listen to your body and adjust the exercises as needed. If you experience any pain or discomfort during the practice, please stop and consult with a healthcare professional. Enjoy your chair yoga routine!

EXERCISE 16: SEATED FORWARD FOLD

Introduction:

The Seated Forward Fold stretches the hamstrings, lower back, and shoulders, promoting flexibility and relaxation.

Instructions:

- ➤ Sit tall on the chair with your feet flat on the floor.
- ➤ Inhale deeply and lengthen your spine.
- ➤ Exhale slowly as you hinge forward from your hips, reaching your hands towards your feet or the floor.
- ➤ Allow your head and neck to relax.
- ➤ Feel the stretch in your hamstrings, lower back, and shoulders.
- ➤ Hold the position for a few breaths.

Benefits:

- ➢ Stretches the hamstrings, promoting flexibility.
- ➢ Relieves tension and tightness in the lower back.
- ➢ Calms the mind and promotes relaxation.

Image: 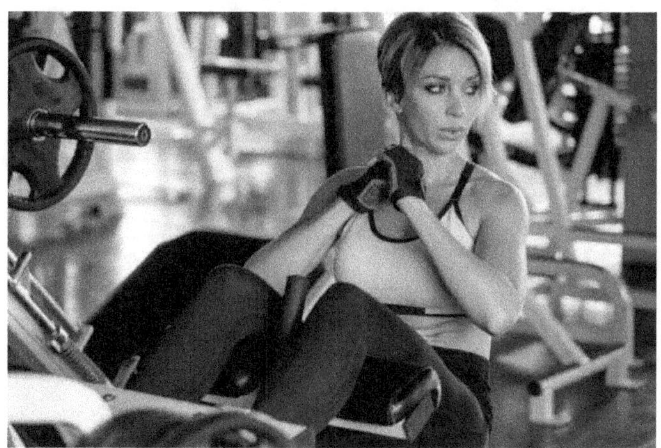

Sets and Repetitions:

Perform 3-5 sets, holding the stretch for 15-30 seconds in each set.

EXERCISE 17: SEATED SHOULDER ROLLS

Introduction:

Seated Shoulder Rolls release tension in the shoulders and upper back, improve posture, and enhance mobility.

Instructions:

- Sit tall on the chair with your feet flat on the floor.
- Inhale deeply and lift your shoulders up towards your ears.
- Exhale as you roll your shoulders back and down, squeezing your shoulder blades together.
- Inhale again and roll your shoulders forward.

Repeat the shoulder rolls, alternating between rolling them back and then forward.

Benefits:

- ➢ Relieves tension and stiffness in the shoulders and upper back.
- ➢ Improves posture and alignment.

Enhances shoulder mobility and range of motion.

Image:

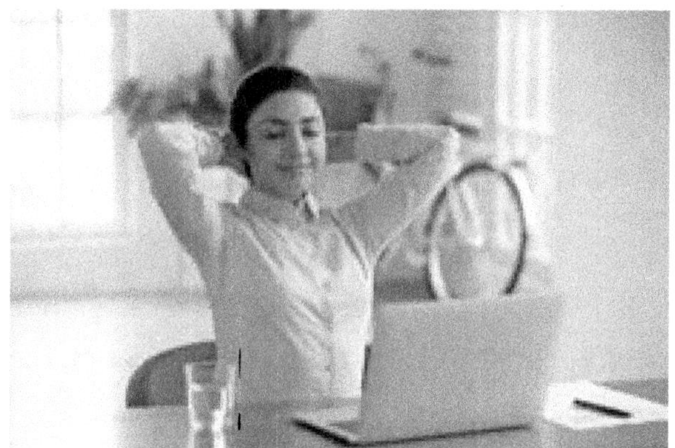

Sets and Repetitions:

Perform 2-3 sets, rolling the shoulders back and forward 8-10 times in each set.

EXERCISE 18: SEATED QUAD STRETCH

Introduction:

The Seated Quad Stretch targets the quadriceps muscles, promoting flexibility and relieving tightness in the front of the thighs.

Instructions:

> ➤ Sit tall on the chair with your feet flat on the floor.
> ➤ Inhale deeply and engage your core.
> ➤ Exhale as you lift your right foot off the floor, bending your knee and bringing your heel towards your gluts.
> ➤ Reach back with your right hand and gently hold on to your right ankle or shin.
> ➤ Feel the stretch in the front of your right thigh.
> ➤ Hold the stretch for a few breaths, then switch sides.

Benefits:

➢ Stretches the quadriceps muscles, improving flexibility.

➢ Relieves tightness and discomfort in the front of the thighs.

➢ Enhances knee and hip joint mobility.

Image:

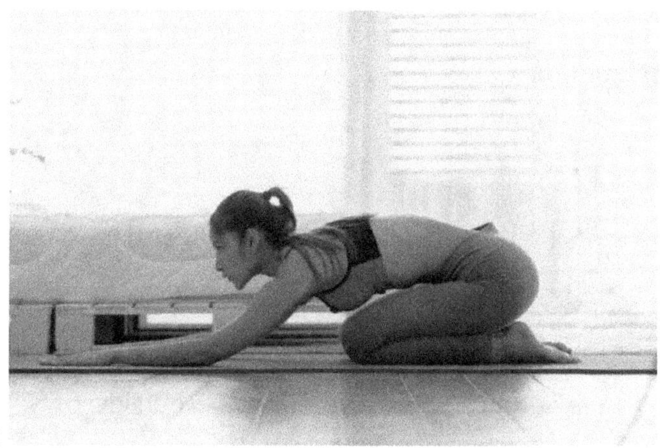

Sets and Repetitions:

Perform 2-3 sets on each side, holding the stretch for 20-30 seconds.

EXERCISE 19: SEATED SPINAL TWIST

Introduction:

The Seated Spinal Twist stretches the spine, hips, and shoulders, improving flexibility and releasing tension.

Instructions:

- Sit tall on the chair with your feet flat on the floor.
- Inhale deeply and lengthen your spine.
- Exhale slowly as you twist your torso to the right, placing your left hand on the outside of your right thigh and your right hand on the back of the chair.
- Gently twist from your waist, keeping your head aligned with your spine.

Feel the stretch along your spine, hips, and shoulders.

Hold the twist for a few breaths, then switch sides.

Benefits:

- ➢ Stretches the spine, hips, and shoulders.
- ➢ Improves spinal mobility and flexibility.
- ➢ Relieves tension and tightness in the upper body.

Image:

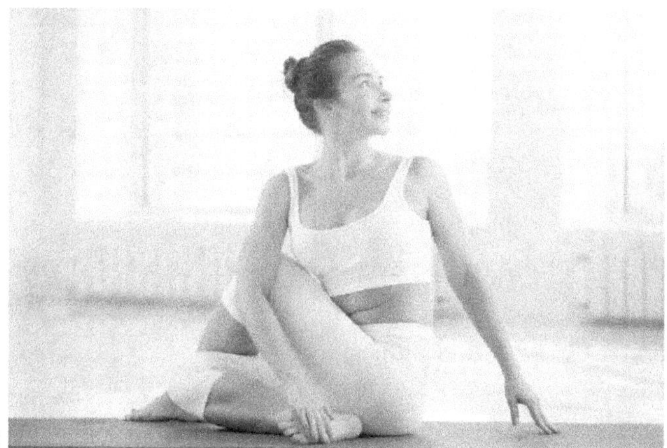

Sets and Repetitions:

Perform 3-5 sets on each side, holding the twist for 3-5 breaths.

EXERCISE 20: SEATED CALF RAISES

Introduction:

Seated Calf Raises strengthen and tone the calf muscles, promoting lower leg stability and balance.

Instructions:

> Sit tall on the chair with your feet flat on the floor.

Inhale deeply and engage your core.

> Exhale as you raise your heels off the floor, lifting your body weight onto the balls of your feet.
> Hold the position for a few seconds, squeezing your calf muscles.
> Inhale as you lower your heels back down to the floor.
> Repeat the calf raises, performing controlled and smooth movements.

Benefits:

> ➢ Strengthens and tones the calf muscles.

> ➢ Improves lower leg stability and balance.

> ➢ Enhances ankle joint strength and mobility.

Image:

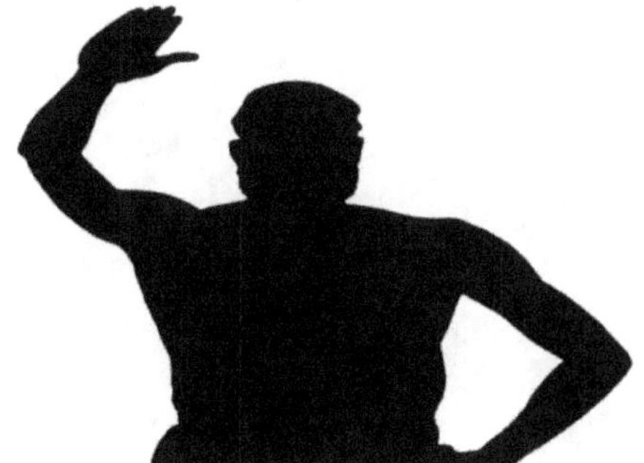

S

Perform 2-3 sets of 10-15 calf raises, gradually increasing the number of repetitions as you build strength.

Remember to listen to your body and adjust the exercises as needed. If you experience any pain or discomfort during the practice, please stop and consult with a healthcare professional. Enjoy your chair yoga routine!

WORKOUT PLAN

40. Each day includes a different exercise to add variety to your routine.

Day	Exercise	Sets and Repetitions
1	Seated Leg Cross Twist	3-5 sets, hold for 3-5 breaths
2	Seated Wrist and Finger Stretch	2-3 sets, hold for 10-15 seconds
3	Seated Hip Opener	2-3 sets, hold for 20-30 seconds
4	Seated Eagle Arms	3-5 sets, hold for 10-15 seconds
5	Seated Abdominal Twist	3-5 sets, hold for 3-5 breaths
6	Seated Forward Fold	3-5 sets, hold for 15-30 seconds
7	Seated Shoulder Rolls	2-3 sets, 8-10 rolls in each set
8	Seated Quad Stretch	2-3 sets, hold for 20-30 seconds

9	Seated Spinal Twist	3-5 sets, hold for 3-5 breaths
10	Seated Calf raises	2-3 sets, 10-15 raises in each set
11	Seated Leg Cross Twist	3-5 sets, hold for 3-5 breaths
12	Seated Wrist and Finger Stretch	2-3 sets, hold for 10-15 seconds
13	Seated Hip Opener	2-3 sets, hold for 20-30 seconds
14	Seated Eagle Arms	3-5 sets, hold for 10-15 seconds
15	Seated Abdominal Twist	3-5 sets, hold for 3-5 breaths
16	Seated Forward Fold	3-5 sets, hold for 15-30 seconds
17	Seated Shoulder Rolls	2-3 sets, 8-10 rolls in each set
18	Seated Quad Stretch	2-3 sets, hold for 20-30 seconds
19	Seated Spinal Twist	3-5 sets, hold for 3-5 breaths
20	Seated Calf raises	2-3 sets, 10-15 raises in each set

CONCLUTION

In conclusion, chair yoga offers a multitude of benefits for women over 40, providing a gentle yet effective form of exercise that can be easily incorporated into daily routines. This practice caters to the specific needs and challenges faced by this age group, promoting flexibility, strength, balance, and overall well-being.

By engaging in chair yoga, women over 40 can experience improved joint mobility, reduced stiffness, and enhanced posture. The exercises target key areas such as the spine, hips, shoulders, and legs, helping to alleviate common discomforts associated with aging. Additionally, chair yoga offers mental and emotional benefits by reducing stress, promoting relaxation, and fostering mindfulness.

One of the remarkable aspects of chair yoga is its accessibility. It can be practiced virtually anywhere, making it an ideal choice for those with limited mobility or who prefer a low-impact exercise option. The support of the chair provides stability and ensures safety during the practice, allowing individuals to focus on their movements and breath without fear of falling or strain.

Furthermore, chair yoga goes beyond the physical realm. It offers an opportunity for self-care, self-reflection, and self-empowerment. By dedicating time to this practice, women over 40 can cultivate a deeper connection with their bodies and develop a sense of inner strength and resilience.

So, to all the inspiring women over 40, I encourage you to embrace chair yoga as a valuable addition to your lifestyle. Take a few moments each day to honor your body, nourish your mind, and uplift your spirit. Celebrate the journey of self-care and personal growth that chair yoga can offer. Remember that it is never too late to embark on a path of wellness and vitality.

Start today and embark on this empowering journey of chair yoga. Embrace the opportunity to prioritize your well-being and experience the transformative effects it can have on your life. Your body, mind, and soul deserve the care and attention that chair yoga provides. Embrace the practice, enjoy the journey, and witness the positive impact it brings to your life.